The Basics of Dry Cupping

Beginners Guide on the Benefits of Dry Cupping with a Simple How-To Guide

MARY CONRAD

ISBN: 1539662551
ISBN-13: 978-1539662556

DEDICATION

This book is for my daughter, Valia, and my supportive husband Vincent. I wouldn't be inspired to write if it wasn't for both of you!

MARY CONRAD

MY OTHER BOOKS

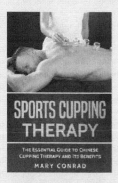

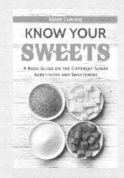

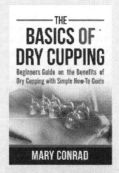

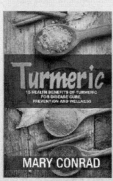

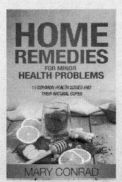

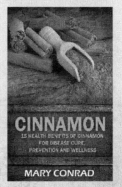

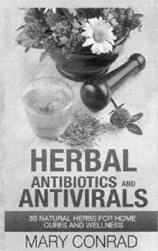

MARY CONRAD

Disclaimer

This book provides general information, personal experiences and extensive research regarding health and related subjects. The information provided in this book, and in any linked materials, is based on my own personal experience and is for informational purposes only. It is not intended to be interpreted as a professional medical advice. Speak with your physician or a trusted healthcare professional prior to taking any nutritional or herbal supplements. Please keep in mind that reactions and results may vary from each individual due to differences in state of health

Before considering any guidance from this book, please ensure you do not have any underlying health conditions, which may interfere with the suggested healing methods. If the reader or any other person has a medical concern or pre-existing condition, please consult with an appropriately licensed physician or healthcare professional. Never disregard professional medical advice or delay in seeking it because of something you have read in this book or in any linked materials.

TABLE OF CONTENTS

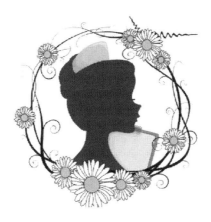

Introduction

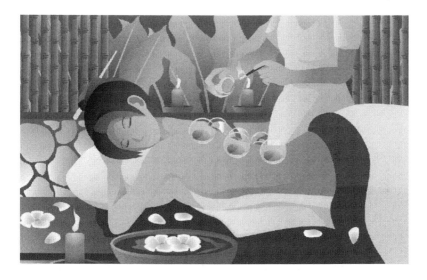

Cupping has been around since ancient times—for about 5,000 years to be exact. It is believed to have originated in Egypt and became popular among the Chinese. Similar to acupuncture and acupressure, it is believed to relieve certain symptoms and conditions when applied to key points in the body. Some of the treatments are mild and cause only mild discomfort whereas there are those that are more serious and applied to a more intense session. It has a wide range of benefits for your health and wellness. Some of these include promoting muscle relaxation and improving immunity.

In this book, you can expect more information on the merits of cupping.

Some of the topics discussed include:

- History of Cupping
- The Basics of the Therapy
- Complementary Treatments for Cupping
- How to Perform Cupping, Both the Old and New Methods
- Reasons to Try Cupping

There's often a reason why alternative therapies are passed on from generation to generation. In a holistic perspective, it is non-invasive with benefits that do not rely on the use of pharmaceuticals medicine. Take a step towards health today and take the wonderful journey with me to discover the wonders of cupping.

.

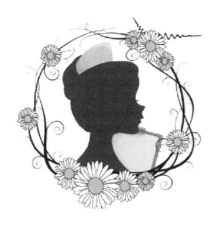

Chapter 1

What is Cupping?

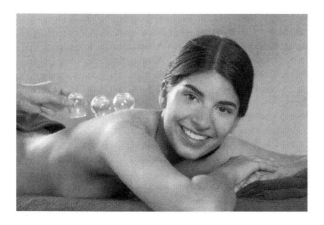

Ventosa, also known as cupping, is a practice where someone places various "cups" on different parts of the body. Using fire or a pump gun, a suction effect is created, raising the skin and drawing the blood to the surface. This is a practice used commonly throughout the Middle East, Europe, and Asia to treat swelling, chronic pain, inflammation, rheumatism, migraines, bronchitis and even the common cold. There are recent studies that suggest it can treat a variety of other ailments as well.

History of Cupping

In the Ebbers Papyrus, all the way from Egypt, you can find the earliest known use of cupping, placing it around 5,000 years old. However, it is also mentioned in Chinese medical treatises that date back about 3,000 years. Hippocrates, a Greek doctor responsible for the Hippocratic Oath, mentions cupping around 400 B.C., and the prophet Mohammad even recommended it in the Quran 1,400 years ago. However, you'll also find it in Finland, where it's been practiced since the 15th century.

It's a popular treatment in Asia, Finland, and the Middle East. However, Americans know very little about cupping, as it is not a common Western medical practice. Cupping goes by many names such as bekam, giac hoi, bag wan, and bentusa in Southeast Asia. In the Middle East, it is commonly referred to as badkesh, hijama, and hejamat. In Chinese hospitals, cupping is considered to be a medical treatment and not classified as alternative medicine.

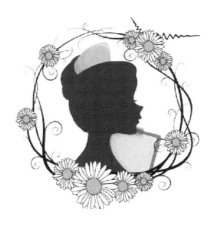

Chapter 2

The Basics of Dry Cupping

Dry cupping is commonly considered as a "warming" treatment. It is performed on intact skin and won't show any signs of bleeding. It can be performed at home with relative ease. Dry static cupping is not complicated and fairly easy. It only requires a little bit of knowledge on where the cups will be placed during different conditions.

Precautions and Contraindications:

First off, the overall health status of the individual must be taken into account. Cupping should not be done to the very young (below 3 years old) and the weak elderly.

For those who are taking anticoagulants, exercise caution when getting this treatment. It would be best to get approval from your physician. The main reason behind this is that cupping could cause excessive bruising and increases the risk of bleeding in the capillaries.

Cupping can't be performed on an empty stomach. It can lead to dizziness and plummets the energy levels of the client. It is best to eat a light meal about an hour and a half prior to the treatment schedule.

If you have any open wounds on the treatment site, cupping is contraindicated. This can lead to infection and further complications. For any condition where the skin integrity is compromised, cupping should not be performed. This includes sunburns, acute stages of inflammation, over fresh scars and burns.

Exercise caution when cupping pregnant women. Use only light to medium cupping up until the sixth month. After which, cupping should be avoided.

Those who have had heart attacks over the last 6 months, can't be treated with cupping. The same goes with those who are in the last stage of cancer (Stage 4: Metastatic Cancer), hemophilia and other blood disorders.

Avoid cupping over moles.

Reminders Prior to Treatment:

Inquire about the individual's pain threshold. This will determine the intensity of the treatment, since it should not be painful for the client. There will be a "pulling" sensation as the cups are placed.

Ensure that area where the procedure will be performed is warm and cozy since the pores will be opened during the treatment. Circulating wind should be avoided, since it is believed that air can cause body pain and discomfort after cupping. Open pores make it easy for wind to enter the pores.

Clean the site where the cups will be placed. This will avoid bacteria from entering the pores during the procedure.

Warm the treatment area. This can be done by massaging using petrissage and effleurage. This helps promote relaxation. Remind the client that staying still during the treatment is important, so as not to dislodge the cups.

For areas with lots of hair, it might be challenging to create an effective suction. Apply oil liberally throughout the area before the session since it can help with this problem.

What to expect throughout the procedure

There are different ways in which cupping will be performed which can either be the traditional fire cupping or the more contemporary vacuum cupping method.

During the fire cupping procedure, the size of the flame is dependent on the strength of the cupping method which can be light, medium or strong. The flaming ball of cotton won't touch the skin. It'll only be used to heat the cups for application. It will be uncomfortable but not painful. Initially, there will be a "pulling" sensation. After a few minutes, there will be small pinpricks of sensation (light pins and needles) where the cups are placed as the fluids under the fascia are drawn to the surface of the skin. The cups can be removed at any time that the client feels too much pain from the procedure. The first treatment will always be short, since the body will require some time to adjust to the treatment.

For vacuum cupping, there are different types of cups used depending on the treatment. For home use, the twist-top cups are popular since they're cheap but effective in providing the necessary suction. It only takes about two full twists to create a light suction, about four to five for medium and between five and up for strong. This may vary according to the individual's pain threshold. Another cup that is commonly used is the pump gun cupping set. This is much more convenient than a twist top and is usually used by professionals since it can easily create suction without as much effort. If the cups are dislodged, you can conveniently reattach the cup on the pump gun and reapply the cups unlike the twist top where you need to twist the knob to the original position prior to reapplying. There's no difference on how the application feels between fire cupping and vacuum cupping. The time frames are also similar for initial treatment and can be stretched out to 30 minutes in follow up sessions.

The bruising or cupping marks begin to form after two minutes of static cupping. The area will feel warm but not painful. The normal bruising appears as small clusters of pinpricks that are red or pink. The bruise will disappear within a week or two.

There are varied reports on how cupping affect different people. It usually depends on the reason they're doing the treatment. For those with muscle problems, the usual feedback after the procedure is that they feel lesser pain in the area and increased mobility. A common side effect is relaxation.

Bruising and Interpretation

There are different ways to interpret cupping marks. For professional TCM practitioners, they can diagnose a condition based on the cupping marks after a session as well as by checking the tongue.

Color	Indications
Pale	Pale – blood or qi deficiency Pale, thin, and dry – blood deficiency Pale and wet – qi deficiency Pale and swollen – qi deficiency Pale, swollen, and wet – yang deficiency
Pink	Normal or just mild disorder
Red	Red – excessive body heat Red and yellow coat – excess heat in the body Red and wet – damp heat Dry and red - injuries
Dark Red	Extreme body heat
Purple	Stagnation Purple and place - cold
Blue	Severe internal cold

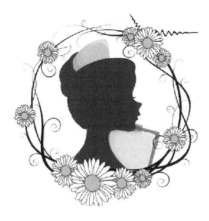

Chapter 3

Traditional Concept of Cupping

The popularity of dry cupping throughout different areas of the East and West stems from a common belief that the **changes in climate or seasons affect the body profoundly**. Some of this true when placed in today's concepts. If you've ever gotten sick each time spring starts, then you've had a firsthand experience on how seasons can cause changes in your health.

The main culprit of in the cause of illness, whether traditional Islamic, Chinese or Ayurverda, is the presence of **WIND** inside the body. The wind is believed to carry diseases as well as cause muscle aches and pains. According to a Buddhist monk, when wind passes through a small opening (such as the pores in the skin), it "pierces the flesh like a dagger", which explains why direct exposure to the air vent or air conditioning can become uncomfortable after a few minutes. The wind enters the body through the pores of the skin, the eyes, ears and head. For the most part, wind affects the upper parts of the body since it is considered as Yang. The opposite of the wind is **DAMP**, which is considered the Yin. It affects the lower portions of the body. This can be observed in the elderly who can often "feel" the signs of rain before it even occurs.

To put things simply, the main reason why folks used cupping throughout history is that it was effective in removing the effects of seasonal and climate changes such as the Hot, Wind and Damp from the muscles and tendons of the body. This in turn removes the pain and improves the mobility of the affected person. Some even claim that it helps increase the rate of recovery from common health issues.

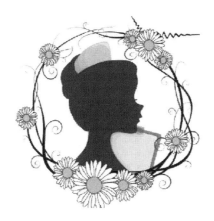

Chapter 4

Cupping Sets

The cupping sets have evolved as the therapy gained more attention and use. The earliest known cupping set was made with animal horns, which were cut at the tip to allow the medicine man or woman to apply manual suction using the mouth. The suction was maintained by covering the hole with a mixture of masticated leaves and saliva that is pushed from the mouth into the hole using the tongue right after manual suction.

The cups then evolved into bamboo, which is still used for herbal cupping, to the more modern ones we enjoy today. The more common sets now are made of glass, plastic and silicone.

CUPPING SETS BASED ON MATERIAL

Glass cupping set:

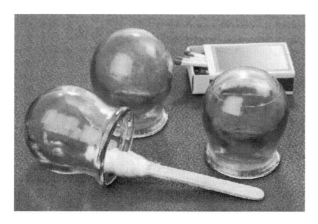

This cupping set is used for the more traditional methods of cupping. It is usually the set of choice for fire cupping since glass can easily hold hot air and provide a good suction. For wet cupping, glass is preferable since it can be sterilized easily to avoid infection.

A glass cupping set can come in different forms. The traditional forms are rounded glass in different sizes. The modern ones are modified with a nozzle at the top where you can attach a pump gun to create a vacuum without the use of fire. Some have modified the set to have a vacuum twist-top nozzle attached into the cup for convenience.

Plastic cupping set:

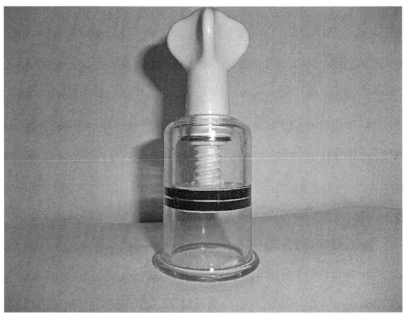

Spequix twist-top cup

Plastic cupping set is commonly used for massage cupping as well as those sets that are sold for home use. These sets are durable, and usually see-through and mimics the form and look of glass cups. The good thing about the cups is they are hard to break. For those who like to do their own cupping therapy at home, there's always a strong chance that you'll drop the cup after putting some oil on the area you want to cup.

Some practitioners may use plastic cups during wet cupping but usually they would likely opt for medical grade glass cups. Plastic cups are usually made with Perspex plastic, which gives off a clean and clear finish that makes it very similar to glass. This can be sterilized as well.

Silicone cupping set:

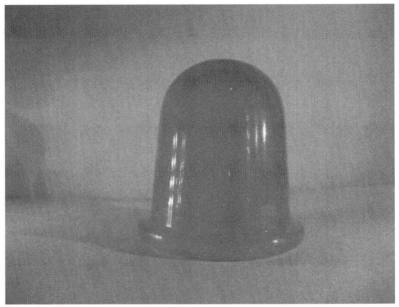

Spequix silicone cup

These are the most durable set around. It's also used for massage cupping. Silicone cups doesn't require heat or any other equipment other than your hand.

To use this cup, you can give it a squeeze to create a vacuum. Place it on the treatment site. You can give the cup an extra squeeze to tighten the vacuum as well as release. You can soak the cups in warm water to soften it if it's too hard. It takes a lot of effort to use these. You'll have to squeeze it each time it pops off the skin to get a proper vacuum. It comes in different forms and sized depending on the treatment site

Rubber cupping set

Rubber cupping sets are similar to silicone sets. The main difference is that rubber tends to wear down faster. These cups are for personal use since it can't be sterilized or cleaned with a strong solution. However, it does provide a good suction and can be used on the soft parts of the body such as the face, stomach and legs.

Bamboo cupping set

This is a common cupping set used in China, mainly due to the ease of use. This set doesn't break easy, doesn't require much in terms of storage and easily available. There are several challenges when using this type of cup. When the bamboo cups are aged, splinters in the rim of the cups may form from minor cracks. This can lead to discomfort during treatment. There's also no way of determining the suction placed on the skin since the cups aren't transparent. This is often the cup of choice for herbal cupping treatment.

CUPPING SETS BASED ON FUNCTION

Magnetic cupping sets

This cupping set comes in two forms: electromagnetic cupping apparatus (ECA) and the squeeze-top magnetic rubber cups.

The magnetic cupping set is said to increase the benefits of cupping, especially when applied to joints such as on the elbows and knees. The ECA is controlled by a machine that adjusts the electromagnetic stimulation as well as the suction. The device is quite bulky and expensive. The treatment is costly and often only offered in Chinese practices. Sterilization is only done occasionally for this device since the cables and the magnets make cleaning difficult.

A cheaper alternative comes in the form of the squeeze-top magnetic cups. It claims to have the same benefits in a more portable form.

MARY CONRAD

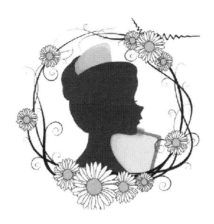

Chapter 5

Dry Cupping Points

F2 – deafness, toothache, sore eyes, arthritis.
F4 – sinusitis, facial paralysis, trigeminal neuralgia, blocked nose
F1 – mouth ulcers, toothache, facial paralysis, jaw problems
N3 – dry mouth, mumps, tonsillitis
TH4 – asthma, cough, bronchitis, pneumonia
TH1 – pharyngitis, bronchitis, asthma, vocal cord problems, hoarse voice
TH6 – jaundice, hepatitis, enlarged liver, gallstones
TH7 – cardiac spasms, heart problems
TH8 – heart valve problems, cardiac spasm
TH2 – insufficient lactation, bronchial spasm, chest pain
A3 – hepatitis, enlarged liver
TH5 – chest pain, ischemia, cardiac spasm
TH2 – chest pain, mastitis, bronchial asthma, insufficient lactation
TH3C – bronchitis, chest pain, bronchial asthma
F3- rhinitis, vertigo, sinusitis, dizziness
HI – migraine, facial paralysis, blurred vision, trigeminal neuralgia, eye pressure
LE15- arthritis

LE14 – itching of the groins, endometriosis

LE6 – knee pain, knee cap problems, knee joint, thigh pain

L13 – liver problems, irregular menstruation, urine incontinence

A7- irregular menstruation, ovarian dysfunction, appendicitis, infertility

LE11 – abnormal uterine bleeding, irregular menstruation, wet dreams, dysmenorrhea

LE12 – irregular menstruation, uterine bleeding, menstrual cramps

LE13 – liver problems, kidney problems, urinary incontinence, irregular menstruation

A8 – endometriosis, irregular menstruation, cystitis, hernia

LE8- uterine bleeding and irregular menstruation

LE7 – knee cap problems, thigh pain, hip pain, knee pain

A4- diabetes, enlarged spleen

A5- kidney stones, constipation, kidney dysfunction, kidney pain

UE3 – shoulder pain

A1 – peptic ulcers, gastritis, bloated stomach, vomiting, indigestion, hiccups

A6- irregular menstruation, appendicitis, vaginal discharge

These cupping points are called Tibb Cupping Points and should only be used if you're using the dry cupping technique.

TIBB CUPPING POINTS

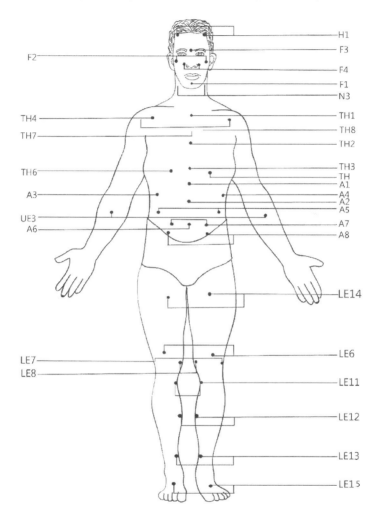

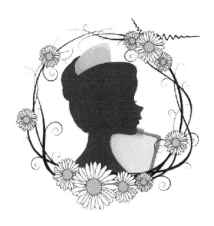

Chapter 6

Hijama Cupping Points

Cupping points help to relieve certain ailments. This is based on the belief that certain points in the body are interconnected, so when an external point is provided treatment, it also treats the internal problem. For muscle pains, this is a more direct therapy that helps the muscles relax, which diminishes most of the discomfort.

Please note that extensive cupping for specific ailments are best done by trained professionals. Always check with your primary physician prior to undergoing any alternative treatment to avoid potential complications. Not all of the points need to be targeted for the treatment to be effective.

Anatomical Cupping Points

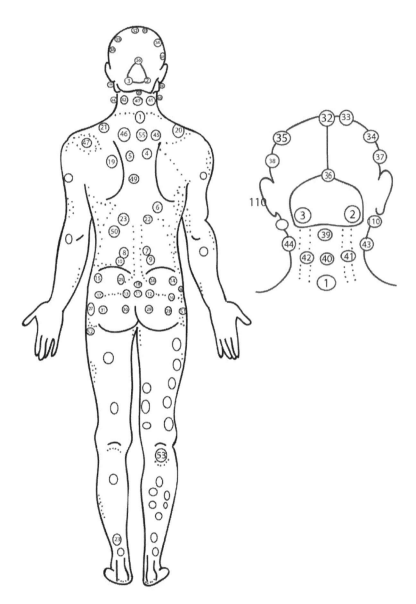

Figure 1.1: Cupping points at the back, including the head

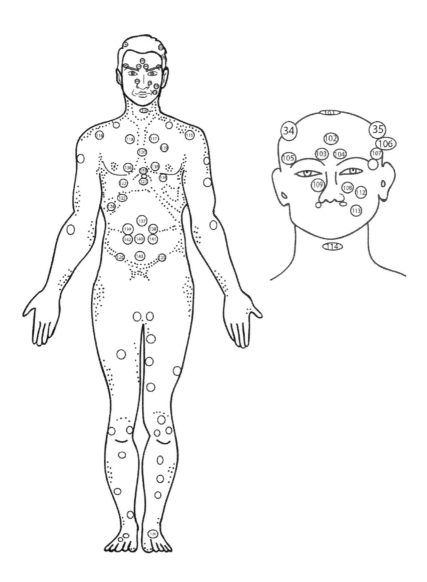

Figure 1.2: Cupping points in the front of the body, including the front of the face.

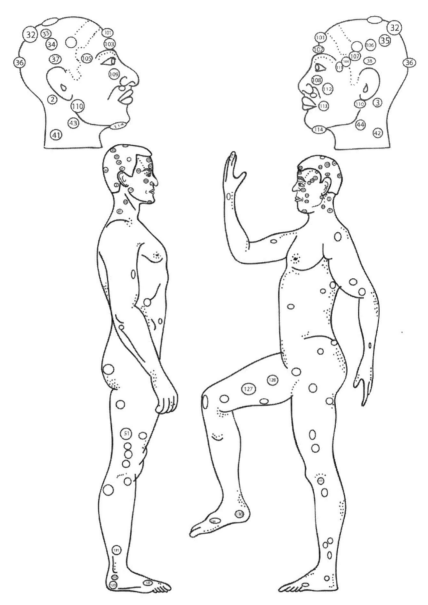

Figure 1.3: Cupping points from the sides of the body including the face

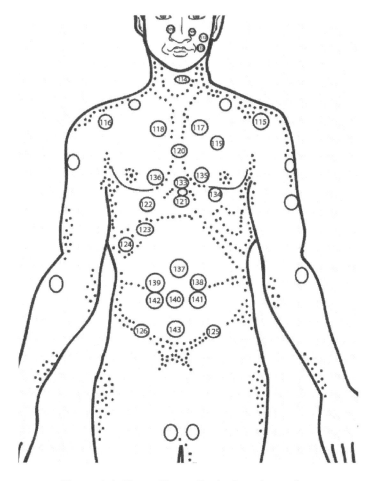

Figure 1.4: Front Upper Body Cupping points

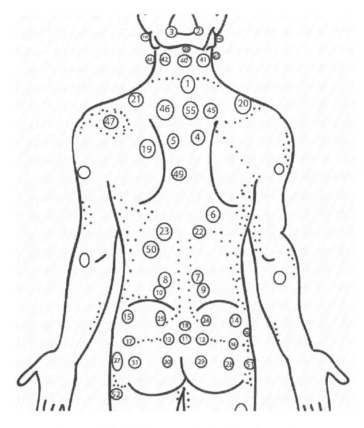

Figure 1.5: Back Upper Body Cupping Points

Note: The numbered circles on the figures indicate specific cupping points while the unnumbered circles are areas which can be cupped for any discomfort in the area but isn't considered as a cupping point.

You can download a PDF copy of the images on www.maryconradrn.com for a full-page copy of the images above. Subscribe to the email list to grab the copy.

HIJAMA CUPPING POINTS		
Ailment	Basic Description	Cupping (Hijama) Points
Rheumatism	Painful joints	1, 55, in addition to all areas of pain
Knee Pain		1, 55, 11, 12, 13 and cupping around the knee and you may add 53, 54
Edema	Swollen tissue due to buildup of fluid	1, 55, 130, the right and left side of the heel and you may add 9, 10
Sciatic pain (Right leg)	Nerve pain from the buttock which goes down the leg	1, 55, 11, 12, 26, 51 and places of pain on the leg especially the beginning and the end of the muscle
Sciatic pain (Left leg)	Nerve pain from the buttock which goes down the leg	1, 55, 11, 13, 27, 52 and places of pain on the leg especially the beginning and the end of the muscle
Back pain		1, 55 and cupping on both sides of the spine and places of pain
Neck/shoulder		1, 55, 40, 20, 21 and

pain		places of pain
Gout	Swollen joints due to excess uric acid	1, 55, 28, 29, 30, 31, 121 and places of pain
Rheumatoid Arthritis		1, 55, 120, 49, 36 and all large and small joints
Hemiplegia	Paralysis of one half of the body	1, 55, 11, 12, 13, 34 or 35 and all the injured joints, massage daily
Quadriplegia	Paralysis of all four limbs	1, 55, 11, 12, 13, 34, 35, 36 and all body joints and daily massage
Immune system deficiency		1, 55, 120, and 49
Muscle spasm		several dry cupping around the affected muscle
Poor blood circulation		1, 55, 11 and ten cups on both sides of the spine from the top to the bottom in addition to taking a teaspoon of pure organic, raw, apple cider vinegar and honey every other day
Tingling arms		1, 55, 40, 20, 21, arm muscles and affected

		joints
Tingling feet		1, 55, 11, 12, 13, 26, 27, feet, joints and affected muscles
Abdominal pain		1, 55, 7, 8 and dry cupping on 137, 138, 139, 140, as well as dry cupping on the back opposite to the pain
Hemorrhoids	Swollen vessels around the anus	1, 55, 121, 11, 6 and dry cupping on 137, 138, 139
Annual Fistula	Opening in the skin near the anus, due to formation of a channel through which fluid leaks	1, 55, 6, 11, 12, 13 and cupping around the anus and above the fistula hole
Prostate and Erectile dysfunction, ED	Male impotence and urinary difficulty due to enlarged prostate gland	1, 55, 6, 11, 12, 13 and you may add for ED 125, 126, 131 on both legs, and dry cupping on 140, 143
Chronic coughs and lung diseases		1, 55, 4, 5, 120, 49, 115, 116, 9, 10, 117, 118, 135, 136, and two cups below both knees
Hypertension	High blood pressure	1, 55, 2, 3, 11, 12, 13, 101, 32, 6, 48, 9, 10, 7, 8, and you may replace

		2, 3 with 43, 44
Stomach problems and ulcers		1, 55, 7, 8, 50, 41, 42 and dry cupping on 137, 138, 139, and 140
Renal (kidney) disease		1, 55, 9, 10, 41, 42 and dry cupping on 137,140
Irritable bowel syndrome	Abdominal cramps and discomfort characterized by bloating and trapped wind and alternating bouts of diarrhea and constipation, often related to anxiety	1, 55, 6, 48, 7, 8, 14, 15, 16, 17, 18, 45, 46 and dry cupping on 137
Chronic constipation	Long term difficulty with opening bowels	1, 55, 11, 12, 13, 28, 29, 30, and 31
Diarrhea		137, 138, 139, and 140
Involuntary urination		After the age of five: dry cupping on 137, 138, 139, 140, 142, 143, 125, and 126
Depression, withdrawal, insomnia	Inability to sleep	1, 55, 6, 11, 32 and below the knees
psychological conditions and nervousness		1, 55, 6, 11, 32 and below the knees
Angiospasm and	Narrowing of the blood	1, 55, 11. Also, cup on

Arteriosclerosis	vessels due to muscular spasm or fatty deposits	the places of pain.
Gastritis	Inflammation in the lining of the stomach	1, 55, and 121
Excessive sleep		1, 55
Food allergies		One dry cup using a light suction directly on the umbilicus pit (belly button)
Sores		1, 55, 129, 120
Heart disease		1, 55, 19, 119, 7, 8, 46, 46, 47, 133, and 134
Diabetes		1, 55, 6, 7, 8, 22, 23, 24, 25, 120, 49
Liver and gall bladder disease		1, 55, 6, 48, 41, 42, 46, 51, 122, 123, 124 and 5 cups on the right, outer leg
Varicose veins	Enlarged, unsightly superficial veins on the legs	1, 55, 28, 29, 30, 31, 132 and around the veins but NOT over the veins
Varicocele	Enlarged unsightly veins on scrotum of male	1, 55, 6, 11, 12, 13, 28, 29, 30, 31, 125, 126
Elephantiasis	Swollen leg due to blockage of lymph channels	1, 55, 11, 12, 13, 120, 49,121 and around the affected leg from the top of the leg to the

		bottom in addition to 125, 126, 53, 54. The patient should rest for 2 days before cupping. He/ She should also raise his/her affected leg up and then place it in warm water for two hours prior to cupping
Skin diseases		1, 55, 49, 120, 129, 6, 7, 8, 11 and cupping on the affected areas
Overweight		1, 55, 9, 10, 120, 49 and areas of desired weight loss), daily massage cupping over area of desired weight loss
Underweight		1, 55, and 121
Cellulite		Daily massage cupping over affected area
Infertility		1, 55, 6, 11, 12, 13, 120, 49, 125, 126, 143, 41, and 42
Thyroid disease		1, 55, 41, and 42
Headaches		1, 55, 2, 3
Migraine	Severe headache associated with nausea	1, 55, 2, 3, 106 and area of pain

	and visual disturbance	
Diseases of the eyes	Retina, eye disorder, blurred vision, atrophy of the eye nerves, glaucoma (Blue Water), cataract (White Water) and weak eye, eye inflammation and secretion of tears and eye sensitivity	1, 55, 36, 101, 104, 105, 9, 10, 34, 35, above the eyebrows and on the hair line above the forehead
Tonsils, throat, gums, teeth, and the middle ear problems	Dizziness, nausea and ringing in ears	1, 55, 20, 21, 41, 42, 120, 49, 114, 43, 44
tinnitus	Weakness of hearing and inflammation of hearing nerve, ringing in the ears	1, 55, 20, 21, 37, 38 and behind the ear
Nasal sinuses		1, 55, 102, 103, 108, 109, 36, 14 and on the hair line
Neuritis	Inflammation of the fifth and seventh nerves	1, 55, 110, 111, 112, 113, 114 and on the affected area
Mute	Unable to speak	1, 55, 36, 33, 107, and 114
To help stop smoking		1, 55, 106, 11, and 32

Convulsion (fits)		1, 55, 101, 36, 32, 107 on sides, 114, 11, 12, 13
Atrophy (loss) of brain cells (oxygen deficiency)		1, 55, 101, 36, 32, 34, 35, and 11 and perform cupping on the joints, muscles and neck, 43 and 44 on the front and back. Perform massage cupping daily
Hemorrhage (vaginal bleeding)		1, 55, and 3 dry cups under each breast daily until bleeding ceases
Amenorrhea	Absence of periods	1, 55, 129, (131 from the outside), 135, 136
Menstruation problems	Painful joints	1, 55 (dry cupping on 125, 126, 137, 138, 139, 140, 141, 142, 143

Table Source: Cupping Resource

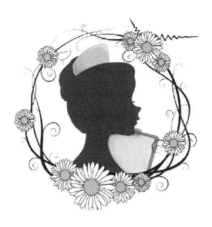

Chapter 7

Different Forms of Cupping

There are alternative ways to perform cupping. It differs with the health condition and the recommendations of the trained professional. These are the different types:

- **<u>Weak Cupping:</u>**

This technique creates a weak or gentle suction when performed. The suction is adjusted either by using a small fire to heat the cups or by adjusting the pump gun. When removed, it leaves a faint circle that won't turn into a bruise.

This cupping method is used to help relax the body and improve blood flow. It helps promote healing by improving the circulation in the body. It can be classified as a light cupping that may be given to patients who are under 7 years old or elderly. The length of the treatment can go as long as 30 minutes. It's recommended for minor health conditions such as colds, asthma, sore throat and tonsillitis.

• Medium Cupping:

Medium cupping is a technique where the suction is slightly stronger than weak cupping. The suction is firm, which is achieved by creating a larger fire to heat the cups. There's a slight discomfort during the treatment and light bruising when the cups are removed.

This is the most common technique used for those with strong chi. It is considered safe for children above 7 years to get this particular treatment. The length of the treatment would be 15 minutes. It can be used for headaches, sports injuries and stress-related conditions.

• Strong Cupping:

This cupping technique is characterized by a strong suction that often drains the chi. This is often used for detoxification and leaves dark bruises after the treatment. According to Chinese medicine, those bruises are actually toxins that are removed from the blood and body. This is the type of cupping that is used for chronic musculoskeletal conditions.

• Moving Cupping/Massage Cupping:

This is the most painful cupping technique among all that is listed. This cupping is performed by using firm suction and manipulating the cups by moving them upwards or downwards on the affected area.

Before the treatment, the back is oiled to lessen the friction and reduce the discomfort of the treatment. One hand is used for moving the cup while the other is placed on the skin right beside it. The hand placed on the skin supports the movement of the cup. The cup should move easily through the skin; if it doesn't, it could mean that the suction is too strong. The treatment should not last longer than five minutes initially, and it isn't recommended for people 16 years old and younger.

- ## Empty/Flash Cupping

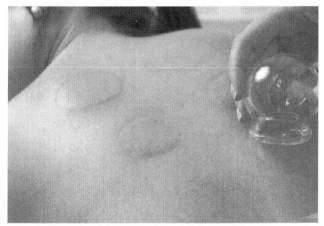

This cupping method is great for children. It is characterized by using medium or strong cupping with short application times. It is applied then removed after a few seconds. It is believed to be helpful for those who have weak chi or energy.

- ## Bleeding Cupping

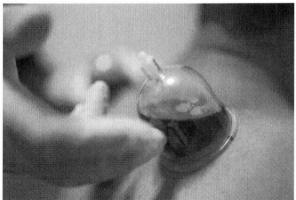

This is the most famous wet cupping technique, mainly due to its popularity in Europe, when it was used as a form of treatment for various health conditions.

The skin is pierced with a lancet prior to the treatment. The bleeding is believed to remove the diseases and toxins that are in the body. This type of cupping is exclusively done by practitioners since the procedure can be risky without proper training.

• **Herbal Cupping**

This is another form of wet cupping that requires a trained practitioner. A prescribed herbal remedy is prepared in a bamboo cup. The cup is placed in a water bath and set to simmer for 30 minutes before application.

This is usually used as a treatment for chronic pain such as those in the joints and knees, as well as conditions caused by the cold, dampness and wind.

• **Water Cupping**

Water cupping is a wet cupping technique that requires a trained and experienced practitioner. It is performed by pouring warm water into the cups about 1/3 of the way. It is then applied to the skin, making sure that none of the water is spilled. This is believed to be effective for asthma, coughs and localized pain.

It's also good to note that cupping differs per country and region. Over time, the practice evolved according to the beliefs and cultural applications of the area. However, the principles behind the practice remains the same.

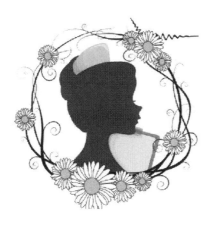

Chapter 8

Vacuum Dry Cupping Procedure

Preparation:

When planning a cupping session, preparation is a must. The cupping set to be used should be clean and placed in a convenient location. The room temperature needs to be warm. The main reason is that during the session, the pores will be opened due to the suction. This makes it easy for wind to enter the body, which can cause more discomfort for the client. Determine the correct cupping points to target during the session. If you feel pain during your session, it is vital that you tell your doctor right away.

The treatment area should be cleaned. This is to avoid bacteria from getting into the open pores. Gently massage the area using petrissage and effleurage to warm it up and relax the client. In a clinic setting, you can expect that the provider would give a detailed explanation about the treatment. For TCM practitioners, they'll perform a general assessment of your health to properly address any issues. A consent form may also be provided for the safety of both parties. For those who want to perform the procedure at home, it is possible.

Reminders for self-cuppers:

- Only perform in areas that you can see and reach.
- Always place your comfort and safety above all else
- Allow your body to adjust to the treatment gradually. This means that you can start at 5 minutes (or less) of static cupping and gradually increase the increments by 2-3 minutes.

Length of the treatment

Initially, a cupping session will last at around 5 minutes on each area. However, this is a baseline time. It also depends on individual tolerance to the treatment. A session can go for 15 minutes to as long as 45 minutes to an hour for trained professionals. For home cuppers, it isn't advised to exceed the 15-minute mark to be on the safe side.

Materials:

- Oil of your choice
- Between 10-20 vacuum cups depending on the area

Procedure:

1. Position the client in a way that is convenient when performing the session.

2. Apply the oil liberally throughout the treatment site.

3. Warm the area through basic massage.

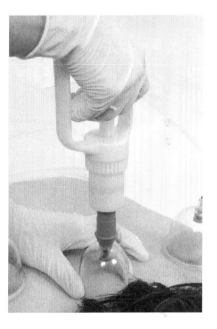

4. Apply the cups on the target cupping points and create a suction either by using a hand-held pump gun, a twist-top vacuum cup or a silicone cup. Use as many cups as necessary to cover the points you need. Also consider the individual's tolerance, since a lot of cups at the same time may not be very comfortable for some.

5. For the initial treatment, use a light to medium cupping method. Determine the tolerance of the client for the pressure and suction and adjust accordingly. In the succeeding sessions, intensity can be increased if well tolerated.

6. After five minutes, remove the cups from the skin. The cups can be placed for up to 15 minutes. Trained professionals can have sessions as long as 40 minutes.

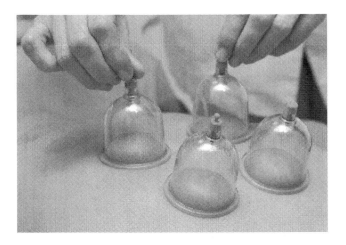

7. Optional: Gently massage the area (effleurage) to help ease the sensation after the skin is released from the suction.

After the procedure:

There are a few reminders after each session.
- Rest is encouraged after the treatment.
- Activities such as running, swimming or working out is not encouraged.
- Avoid exposure to cold and wind

Expect that there will be some marks left by the treatment. The longer the cups are placed on the skin, the more pronounced the mark. However, this is also dependent on the intensity of the cupping procedure. The greater the intensity the darker the marks. The area shouldn't be tender or sore despite the coloration. It will often look a lot worse than the area actually feels. Some practitioners will insist on a back rub, but not every doctor will. It is natural to experience tingling after a session, and this can last from a few minutes to a few hours depending upon the person. For some ailments, such as joint problems, you may be asked to come in more than once. However, two sessions are often the most that you'll get in a week. Most practitioners will want the bruising to be completely gone before you come in again.

Note: *The frequency of the cupping treatment often differs. It depends on the specific effect you want to achieve or the treatment plan that you're given by a professional. For mild cupping in a healthy individual as a form of stress relief and relaxation, it can be performed successively. However, in most cases when a cupping session applies medium to hard cupping techniques, professionals would often wait for a day or two for the bruises to fade before continuing the treatment.*

It's always a good idea to stay on the safe side and allow your body a bit of time to recover from the previous session.

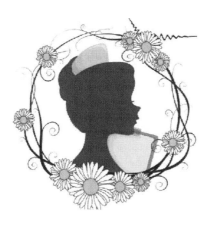

Chapter 9

Moving Cupping

(Massage Cupping)

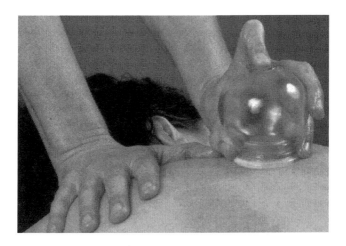

Massage cupping is a form of deep tissue massage that doesn't facilitate the use of hands and instead uses a cup and a pump gun or a massage cup with a built-in vacuum twist-top nozzle to achieve the therapeutic effect. While Chinese cupping is often static with the typical application time of 10-15 minutes, massage cupping allows the movement of the cups with a limited static time of 3 minutes on different cupping points.

The point of this therapy is to get the blood flowing and unblock the lymphatic system. It works by drawing up stagnant blood from the tissues and moving it to the natural exit points in the body. The lymphatic system is then activated and will help by mobilizing the waste for excretion from the body.

Typically, massage cupping can be used together with manual manipulation to achieve an increase in the range of motion, especially for burn victims. For athletes, it can help by relaxing the deep tissues and assists excreting any build-up of lactic acid which causes muscle pain. However, specific treatments are more effective when done by a trained professional.

Here are the steps to performing massage cupping.

Materials:
- cupping set with pump gun or twist-top cups
- therapeutic oil

1. Ask the client to lie down on a flat surface. It can be massage bed or any comfortable bed that encourages relaxation and is convenient for the procedure.

2. Lightly spread oil on the target area. It's preferable to use therapeutic oils that assists the therapeutic effect. The oil will help by making it easier to move the cups.

3. Prepare the clean cups close to the bed. Usually, only one cup is used at a time but it may vary in size depending on the treatment site.

4. Place the cup on the specific cupping point. If you're using a

cupping set with a pump gun and a hose, attach the hose to both the cup and pump gun. This cupping set is more convenient for massage cupping since it's more continuous. When the cup pops off during the massage you can easily pump it up to restore the vacuum. However, you can use any cupping set you have on hand.

5. Create a vacuum using the pump gun to secure the cup. For cupping sets with a vacuum nozzle, just twist it clockwise to create a vacuum and twist counterclockwise to release.

6. Ensure that the vacuum is comfortable and not painful. Slowly move the cups in an outward motion either away from the center of the body or towards the lower extremities. If you encounter areas where the cup won't move, don't force it. For certified practitioners, these stops are often a signal that there's some congestion in the area and extra work needs to be done for those. The skin in the cup is assessed before proceeding. Continue the massage between 5 to 10 minutes for the first session.

Release the suction by pressing right below the rim of the cup for pump gun cupping sets. Massage cupping usually doesn't leave any bruises since it never stays in place for long. However, it may depend on the condition of the client as well as the practitioner who is administering the therapy

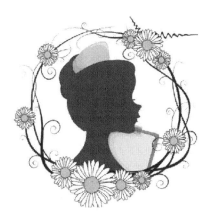

Chapter 10

Traditional Cupping

(Fire Cupping)

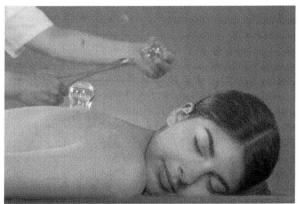

Traditional cupping in Southeast Asia involves the use of fire. It's very similar to Chinese cupping, with only minor differences. The materials used are normally things used around the house. With some help, it can be safely done at home.

Materials:

- Cotton balls
- Coins
- Glass cups
- Alcohol
- Candle
- Match sticks
- Massage Oil

Procedure:

1. Once the materials are ready, the client is asked to remove any clothing that covers the area where the cupping will be performed. In choosing the area, it's often emphasized that the treatment should not be done in bony areas and hairy parts of the body. This is to avoid any discomfort from the suction and possible burning of body hair.

2. Oil is applied on the area for relaxation.

3. The cotton is dipped lightly in alcohol and set aside for later.

4. A coin is then placed on the skin and topped with the cotton ball.

5. Using a match, the cotton is ignited then immediately covered with the glass. This extinguishes the flame right away and results in a vacuum, creating a suction.

6. The cups are left on the skin for five to ten minutes to yield the health benefits. The procedure is repeated in other areas of the body.

Today, the cup is normally heated using a lit cotton ball before application. It reduces anxiety for those who are getting the treatment, and also lowers the risk of minor burns. Below is a simple diagram on how modern fire cupping is performed.

.

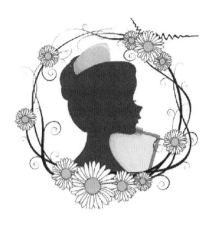

Chapter 11

Alternative Therapies that Go with Cupping

Cupping and Acupuncture

Stick to a basic massage if you don't like needles because acupuncture is a common combination with cupping. In certain practices, such as cupping in Chinese medicine, they're done in tandem. However, historical texts state that cupping was once its own practice, and so they do not always have to go together.

By the Tang Dynasty, around 618-907 A.D., acupuncture was frequently added to cupping. The patient would undergo cupping first before needles were placed on acupuncture points, and then heated bamboo tubes would often be placed over the needles. This made the acupuncture work faster as well as reach deeper. However, this isn't often practiced today. A Chinese clinic will often still recommend acupuncture and cupping together. This is, however, not usually at the same time. The needles will be brought out once you've been cupped, and while the area is still bruised and tingling, the acupuncture is known to hurt a lot less. There are also practitioners that perform needle cupping where cupping is done over acupuncture points while the needle is still in place.

Sometimes, you will experience acupuncture with electrodes that deliver an electrical charge through into your body. This is known to hurt, but it makes the acupuncture work deeper. There is also moxibustion. *Jiu* is the Chinese word for moxibustion, and it involves heat as well as mugwort with traditional acupuncture needles.

About Moxibustion

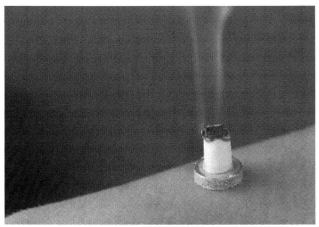

Moxibustion is created by taking mugwort, drying it out and letting it age properly, and pounding it into a mold. One end is set on fire, which will burn slowly to the other end in the same fashion that a cigar does. The mold is a tubular one, and it is wrapped in paper so that it burns slowly, and the paper will flake off as it burns. It'll produce medicinal smoke, but it is less fragrant than incense. There are three ways moxibustion is applied.

- **Direct Scarring:** This is done by making a small cone using the dried mugwort. It is then placed directly on the skin, and the tip is lit and then blown out. It'll singe the skin like incense until it blisters, and this is often done after cupping to help mitigate the pain.

- **Direct Non-Scarring:** This is done nearly the same as direct scarring, except that the mugwort is actually removed before it burns the skin. This gives it no time to form a blister and make a permanent scar.

- **Indirect Moxibustion:** This involves the tubular mold, placing it at acupressure points. It can also be where you place the needles first and the mugwort on top of them, lighting them and then blowing them out. The needle is heated, and it will carry the heat into you while avoiding a direct burn. Electrifying the needles is actually a modern alternative to moxibustion.

Moxibustion is used to treat hypertension, sore muscles, stroke, constipation, cramps and even menstrual pain. The smell it produces will help to stimulate blood circulation to the pelvic area and uterus.

This may be used together with cupping. The process usually utilizes a small moxa, just like on the image above. The burning moxa is placed on the target area and covered with a cup. It's left on the skin for a few minutes, and then removed by the practitioner. This type of cupping requires a trained professional.

Cupping and the Massage "Tui Na"

Tui na is a type of massage that is often done after cupping. *Tui* means "to push," and *na* means "to grasp, squeeze or lift." It is a form of massage that is commonly used after a patient goes through a cupping session. However, it is done before an acupuncture session is scheduled. It is referred to as acupressure because it concentrates on acupoints. This type of massage will rarely use any ointment or oils.

Where It Came From

In Chinese medicine, it is based on the idea of symmetry and balance, and it is meant to help the energy streams flow unobstructed along the meridians. These energy streams are known as *chi*, and in Chinese medicine, it is believed that if chi is blocked, there is an imbalance in the body that needs to be corrected. This can cause illness in the area where the chi is blocked and unable to flow through. Acupressure seeks to open up these blocked passages, restoring the body to its proper balance and harmony.

Why It's Used with Cupping

This practice is used primarily with cupping because if a cupping bruise, say on your lower back, comes out very dark and nearly black, then it will tell the practitioner that there is an imbalance in your lower back. This will help them to know where the chi is blocked. The practitioner should know where they should be concentrating to make sure that you walk out of the practice healthy and happy.

This does not mean that the practitioner will only focus on that one area, though. Doing so could cause a significant imbalance which would block chi in another area. Both sides of the body will still need to be massaged equally, allowing for the chi to flow smoothly. In this practice, it is believed that there are eight defensive gates—areas between each joint—and none should be blocked for optimal health.

It can cause physical, emotional, and even mental illness. It can be anything from an injury or depression. When used with cupping, this method can be directed more efficiently to help make sure that you have a better range of motion, gotten rid of stiff joints, don't suffer from muscle cramps, and enjoy a more stable emotional wellbeing.

Gua Sha and Cupping

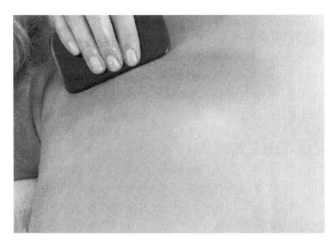

Gua Sha can often be done in tandem with cupping. Gau Sha means scraping, and it's where oil is put over the skin before it is scraped with a coil, rhino horn scraper, ceramic spoon, jade or another traditional object. This can be used to treat sore muscles, exhaustion, cellulite, fever, and general tenderness. No matter what is being used, the skin is being scraped along meridian points. These are where your acupuncture points are as well.

When it is a case of excessive flab, a patient will be told to lie on their back while the doctor scrapes the thighs or tummy towards the groin. This is believed to loosen the fat toward excretory organs so that it can be released later. Gua Sha is known to cause soreness, and it is not uncommon to have bright red scratch marks. These will fade after two to four days in most cases. When used in combination with cupping, the scratches will often fade at the same rate that the bruises do.

It is important to remember that Gua Sha hasn't been proven to be effective. However, many people swear by it. When it is performed properly, the equipment is sterilized and it is meant to be relaxing. The time that Gua Sha is not relaxing is often when it is used in tandem with cupping, as it can produce an acute soreness. It is also not usually seen as relaxing when it's used to treat excessive fat.

When used to treat muscle fatigue, it is often used with a solution of ginger root soaked in vinegar or rice wine. It is an odd treatment, but it is meant to rejuvenate and relax you. Many people will continue to swear by this treatment despite it not being proven effective. No matter if you're having Gua Sha on its own or if you're looking to have it done in tandem with cupping, you need to make sure that you are only being treated by a professional who keeps their equipment sterile at all times.

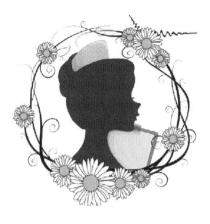

Chapter 12

Benefits of Cupping

There are many reasons that you should try cupping today, but the main one is that when done by a practitioner, it is highly beneficial. It can help manage pain relief and alleviate stress. There are many different types of cupping and activities that can be used in tandem with cupping. Find a practitioner who you're comfortable with and is trained to provide the different complementary treatments. You can say no to something you are uncomfortable with, so never let your fear of one practice that is used in tandem with cupping to stop you from trying the practice as a whole. It is recommended that you try first try cupping from trained practitioner before doing it at home.

Reason #1: Pain Relief

Cupping has been proven to provide some pain relief. This is specific to muscular and at times joint and ligament pain. This is due to cupping softening the tissue with the applied pressure to stagnant areas, increasing the blood flow which will allow for essential nutrients as well as oxygen to get to the tissue.

It can even help as an alternative method to pain relief in cancer patients when coupled with other treatments. Please note that the cupping isn't applied on any visible inflammation or nodes. The cups are for muscle pain experienced during the treatment for cancer. However, any form of cupping is not advised for those who are on the last stage of cancer (Stage 4: Metastatic), since it can enhance the progression of the cancer. Those who are feeling weak are also not advised to undergo cupping.

For those in the healing stages of an injury, the heat, pressure, and suctioning near the site will also allow the unblocking of chi and may increase your energy.

Reason #2: Promote Relaxation

Even if you don't buy into the idea of cupping to help in a physical sense regarding illness and pain, cupping has proven to be relaxing. Chronic stress and mental fatigue can lead to anxiety and depression. It is important to take time to relax and relieve the tension that accumulates in your day-to-day life. Cupping is a great way to do so. This is especially true with massage cupping, which has similar benefits to massage in terms of relaxation.

Reason #3: Relieves Cough, Allergy, and Cold Symptoms

Cupping helps to stimulate vital organs, including the lungs, which will help to speed up healing, clear out phlegm, and even relieve allergy symptoms. It can improve your immune function due to the blood and lymphatic fluid through the body properly. Cupping was primarily used to treat respiratory conditions, including pulmonary tuberculosis and asthma before people had ready access to prescriptions.

When cupping is applied to different points in the body, it can address issues such as congestion and coughing.

Reason #4: Quickens the Healing Process

Cupping is proven to help heal injuries more quickly because it reduces inflammation. Too much inflammation is a bad thing, as it'll lead to health concerns. However, a little inflammation can go a long way in helping quicken the healing process of both injuries as well as illnesses. Blood is drawn up to the affected areas, this not only draws stagnant fluids between the tissues, but it also helps nutrient-rich blood to assist in healing the affected area.

Reason #5: Detoxify the Body

Cupping can also help to release toxins that build up in tissues due to the promotion of better circulation. It will help to improve stagnation, as blood from the affected area are drawn towards the surface of the skin for elimination. This will remove dead cells, toxins, and debris. The toxins are then excreted by the lymphatic system, which is activated in the process of cupping.

Reason #6: Helps Skin Conditions

Cupping can help treat numerous skin conditions as well, including eczema, acne, herpes breakouts, cellulite, and skin inflammation. However, in the process of removing acne, the area is usually nicked to remove the breakout through a cupping session where it opens up the pores. This particular treatment requires professional assistance to avoid complications. Open wounds can lead to infection. It is best to ensure that the items being used is sterile.

Cellulite is a common skin condition among women. Cupping helps with this by increasing the local metabolism in the area and increasing circulation. This is manifested by a tightening of the skin in the affected area after several sessions, which in turn reduces the appearance of cellulite.

Reason #7: Anti-Aging Effect

Cupping is also known to help with anti-aging effects, as it'll help to combat wrinkles that accumulate during the aging process. Your circulation slows down as you age, but cupping improves circulation, allowing more essential nutrients and oxygen to get to your skin. This increases collagen production, ensuring that you have healthier skin while aging naturally.

Reason #8: Helps Digestive Disorders

Cupping is known to help with digestive disorders due to the reduction of symptoms. It can lower the stress response, which is linked to digestive functioning. Frequently throughout the history of cupping, it has been used to treat diarrhea, acute gastritis, loss of appetite, water retention and frequent stomach pains.

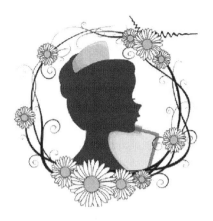

Chapter 13

Getting Rid of the Bruise

The cupping marks or bruise can be bothersome to look at but for practitioners it is a way of looking into your health status. The marks are visible signs of accumulated waste products between the tissues. Since the toxins are drawn out of the tissues, it will be easier for the body to remove it. Normally, a mark will disappear after 3-15 days depending on the form of cupping used.

Cupping marks or bruise isn't an actual bruise, since it is not a result of an injury towards the blood vessel. The marks are just from the fluids moving from the tissues towards the surface of the skin.

There are ways to increase the rate of recovery and encourage the breakdown of the accumulated fluids.

1. Massage the marks in a circular motion. Start from the middle of the mark and work your finger outwards. Do this for 2 minutes with an interval of 2 minutes rest in between. You can do this a few times to lighten dark marks.
2. Apply cabbage juice on the area and gently knead it into the skin.
3. After a session, rehydrate with lots of fluids (water or infused water). This will hasten the elimination of the toxins in the skin.

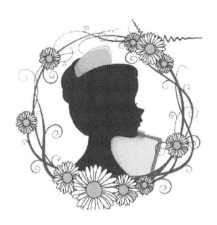

Conclusion

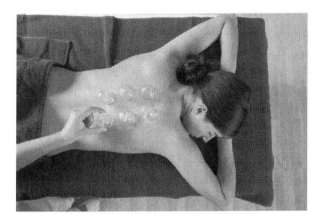

Cupping is a wonderful way to relieve stress, anxiety, and depression, and to relieve pain and promote a healthier, happier you. There is no reason to refrain from cupping. It is always recommended that you see a licensed practitioner to get the most out of your cupping session, but many cupping sets are available for stress and relaxation as well. Cupping is a great way to enhance your life and promote mental and physical health. Try cupping today, and you won't be sorry you did. It is an ancient tradition that has been enriching the lives of those who have used it over the years, whether it is in a spa or as an alternative treatment.

Finally, if you enjoyed this book, then I'd like to ask you for a favor. Would you be kind enough to leave a review for this book on Amazon? It'd be greatly appreciated!

Follow me on Facebook (Mary Conrad) and Twitter (@authormconrad).

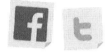

Subscribe to my newsletter to get updates on my latest book and free giveaways!
www.maryconradrn.com

If you have any suggestions or specific natural remedies that you want to have researched and written, shoot me an email at authormaryconrad@gmail.com. I'm always on the lookout for great new topics to write about. :)

Have a great day!

Thank you for taking this journey with me, and good luck!

Author Biography

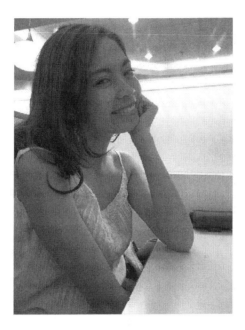

Mary Conrad is a Registered Nurse, who has a strong interest in natural remedies. As a mother, she believes in a holistic approach to health and well-being. Even though she graduated in the health profession, which usually advocates pharmaceutical medication, she believes that prevention is the best step towards health. Backed with scientific research, she wrote these books for both personal information and for others who share the same passion for holistic wellness. It's all about knowing the best natural ways to prevent disease and remedy current health problems. Like every health care provider, she believes in doing no harm, and promoting health. Take a step towards health, and towards nature.

CHECK OUT MY OTHER BOOKS:

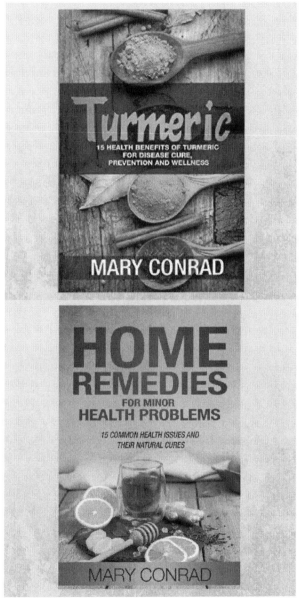

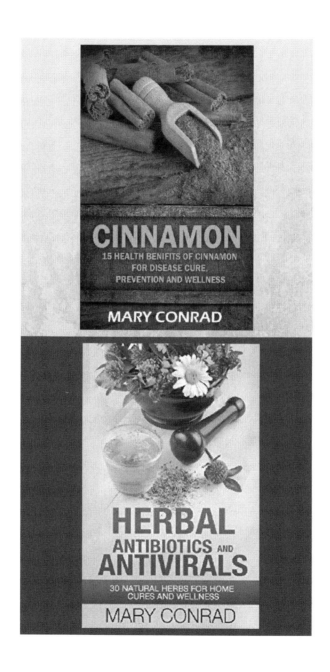

Made in the USA
Columbia, SC
05 November 2019